Keto Slow Cooker Cookbook For Everyone

An Amazing Guide With the Most Wanted Healthy And Tasty Slow Cooker Recipes For Your Ketogenic Diet

Sharon Scott

Disclaimer Notice:

Please note the information contained within this document is for educational and entertainment purposes only. All effort has been executed to present accurate, up to date, and reliable, complete information. No warranties of any kind are declared or implied. Readers acknowledge that the author is not engaging in the rendering of legal, financial, medical or professional advice. The content within this book has been derived from various sources. Please consult a licensed professional before attempting any techniques outlined in this book.

By reading this document, the reader agrees that under no circumstances is the author responsible for any losses, direct or indirect, which are incurred as a result of the use of information contained within this document, including, but not limited to, errors, omissions, or inaccuracies.

Table of Content

Introduction

Thank you for purchasing **Keto Slow Cooker Cookbook For Everyone: An Amazing Guide With the Most Wanted Healthy And Tasty Slow Cooker Recipes For Your Ketogenic Diet**

Cooking with a slow cooker, even though the times are obviously long, so much that it can take up to 10 hours for the most complex preparations, is very simple. Generally speaking, even the most modern models are limited to only two settings, that of time and temperature.

Usually the latter is chosen among three options, low, medium or high and in some cases there is also a "keep warm" button to keep food warm. Obviously the more we set the temperature high, the less time it will take to cook our food.

Speaking of costs, for a slow cooker you do not have to spend a fortune. On the market there are in fact even cheap and good brand around 50/60 dollars. We don't have to worry about spending on electricity, since despite the long cooking times, these products are designed not to consume large amounts of energy. The real big limitation is instead the size, which can make it difficult to place this product in smaller kitchens.

Breakfast Recipes

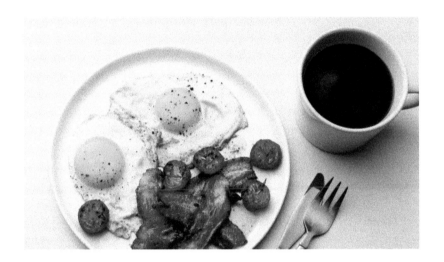

Baked Omelet with Bacon

Preparation Time: 5 minutes

Cooking Time: 30 minutes

Servings: 1

Ingredients:

- 4 eggs
- 140 g diced bacon
- 85 g butter
- 60 g fresh spinach
- 1 tbsp. l finely chopped fresh onions (to taste)
- salt and pepper

Directions:

1. Preheat the oven to 400 ° F. Oil one small baking dish (per serving).

2. Fry the bacon and spinach in the remaining oil.

3. In another bowl, whisk the eggs until it's foamy. Mix the bacon and spinach, gradually adding the fat remaining after frying the products.

4.   Then add finely chopped onions. Flavor the dish with salt and pepper.

5.   Put the mixture into a baking sheet then bake for at least 20 minutes or until golden brown.

6.   Recover the dish and let it cool for a few minutes. After that, you can serve.

Nutrition: Carbohydrates: 12 g Fats: 72 g Proteins: 21 g Calories: 737

Eggplant Pate with Breadcrumbs

Preparation Time: 27 minutes

Cooking time: 6 hours

Servings: 15

Ingredients:

- 5 medium eggplants

- 2 sweet green pepper

- 1 cup bread crumbs

- 1 teaspoon salt

- 1 tablespoon sugar

- ½ cup tomato paste

- 2 yellow onion

- 1 tablespoon minced garlic

- ¼ chili pepper

- 1 teaspoon olive oil

- 1 teaspoon kosher salt

- 1 tablespoon mayonnaise

Directions:

1. Peel the eggplants and chop them.

2.   Sprinkle the chopped eggplants with the salt and let sit for 10 minutes.

3.   Meanwhile, combine the tomato paste with the kosher salt and sugar.

4.   Add minced garlic and mayonnaise. Whisk carefully. Then, peel the onions and chop.

5.   Spray the slow cooker bowl with the olive oil. Add the chopped onions.

6.   Strain the chopped eggplants to get rid of the eggplant juice and transfer the strained eggplants into the slow cooker bowl as well. After this, add the tomato paste mixture.

7.   Chop the chili pepper and sweet green peppers and add them to the slow cooker too. Stir the mixture inside the slow cooker carefully and close the lid.

8.   Cook the dish for 6 hours on LOW. When the time is done, transfer the prepared mix into a bowl and blend it until smooth with the help of the hand blender.

9.   Sprinkle the prepared plate with the bread crumbs. Enjoy!

Nutrition: calories 83, fat 1, carbs 14, protein 18

Keto Omelet with Mushrooms

Preparation Time: 5 minutes

Cooking Time: 10 minutes

Servings: 1

Ingredients:

- 3 eggs

- 30 g butter for frying

- 30 g (60 ml) grated cheese

- 1⁄5 onion

- 3 pcs. mushrooms

- salt and pepper

Directions:

1. Break the eggs then put the contents into a small bowl.

2. Add salt and pepper to taste.

3. Beat the eggs with a fork until a uniform foam is formed.

4. In a pan, heat a piece of butter, and as soon as the butter has melted, pour the egg mixture into the pan.

5.   When the mixture begins to harden and fry, and the eggs on top will still be liquid, sprinkle them with cheese, mushrooms, and onions (to taste).

6.   Take a spatula and gently pry the edges of the omelet on one side, and then fold the omelet in half. As soon as the dish begins to take a golden brownish tint, remove the pan from the stove then place the omelet on a plate.

Nutrition: Carbohydrates: 5 g Fats: 44 g Proteins: 26 g Kcal: 649

Red Beans with the Sweet Peas

Preparation Time: 21 minutes

Cooking time: 6 hours

Servings: 5

Ingredients:

- 1 cup red beans, dried

- 3 chicken stock

- 3 tablespoon tomato paste

- 1 onion

- 1 teaspoon salt

- 1 chili pepper

- 1 teaspoon sriracha

- 1 tablespoon butter

- 1 teaspoon turmeric

- 1 cup green peas

Directions:

1.   Soak the red beans in water for 8 hours in advance.

2.   After this, strain the red beans and put them in the slow cooker.

3.   Add the chicken stock, salt, and turmeric.

4. Close the slow cooker lid and cook the red beans for 4 hours on HIGH.

5. Meanwhile, peel the onion and slice it. Combine the sliced onion with the tomato paste, sriracha, and butter. Chop the chili pepper and add it to the onion mixture.

6. When the time is done, open the slow cooker lid and add the onion mixture.

7. Stir it very carefully and close the slow cooker lid. Cook the dish for 1 hour more on Low.

8. Stir the red beans mixture carefully again and add the green peas. Cook the dish on LOW for 1 more hour. After this, stir the dish gently and serve. Enjoy!

Nutrition: calories 190, fat 3, carbs 18, protein 11

Sandwiches With Salad

Preparation Time: 5 minutes

Cooking Time: 0 minutes

Servings: 1

Ingredients:

- 50 g Roman salad

- 15 g Butter

- 30 g Cheese of Eden cheese or other cheese (to your taste)

- 0.5 pcs Avocado

- 1 pc cherry tomato

Directions:

1. Rinse the lettuce leaves thoroughly and use them as a base for the filling.

2. Oil the leaves, chop the cheese, avocado, and tomato and place on the leaves.

Nutrition: Fats: 34 g Proteins: 10 g Carbohydrates: 3 g Calories: 374

Lunch Recipes

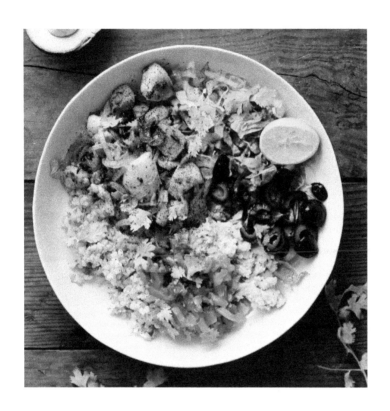

Pulled Pork Salad

Preparation time: 15 minutes

Cooking time: 8 hours

Servings: 4

Ingredients:

- 1 avocado, chopped

- 1 tomato, chopped

- 1 cup lettuce, chopped

- 1 tablespoon olive oil

- ½ teaspoon chili flakes

- 7 oz. pork loin

- 1 cup water

- 1 bay leaf

- 1 teaspoon salt

- ¼ teaspoon peppercorns

Directions:

1. Place the pork loin in the slow cooker.

2. Add the water, bay leaf, salt, and peppercorns.

3. Add the chili flakes and close the lid.

4. Cook the pork loin for 8 hours on Low.

5. Meanwhile, mix the chopped avocado, tomato, and lettuce in a large salad bowl.

6. When the pork loin is cooked, remove it from the water and place it in a separate bowl.

7. Shred the pork loin with two forks.

8. Add the shredded pork loin into the salad bowl.

9. Stir the salad gently and sprinkle with the olive oil.

10. Enjoy!

Nutrition: Calories: 302g, Fat: 22g, Carbs: 5g,Protein: 34g,

Nutritious Lunch Wraps

Preparation time: 20 minutes

Cooking time: 4 hours

Servings: 5

Ingredients:

- 7 oz. ground pork

- 5 tortillas

- 1 tablespoon tomato paste

- ½ cup onion, chopped

- ½ cup lettuce

- 1 teaspoon ground black pepper

- 1 teaspoon salt

- 1 teaspoon sour cream

- 5 tablespoons water

- 4 oz. Parmesan, shredded

- 2 tomatoes

Directions:

1.   Combine the ground pork with the tomato paste, ground black pepper, salt, and sour cream. Transfer the meat mixture to the slow cooker and cook on HIGH for 4 hours.

2.   Meanwhile, chop the lettuce roughly. Slice the tomatoes.

3.   Place the sliced tomatoes in the tortillas and add the chopped lettuce and shredded Parmesan. When the ground pork is cooked, chill to room temperature.

4.   Add the ground pork in the tortillas and wrap them. Enjoy!

Nutrition:

Calories 318,

Fat 7,

Fiber 2,

Carbs 3.76,

Protein 26

Lunch Chicken Wraps

Preparation time: 18 minutes

Cooking time: 6 hours

Servings: 6

Ingredients:

- 6 tortillas

- 3 tablespoon Caesar dressing

- 1-pound chicken breast

- ½ cup lettuce

- 1 cup water

- 1 oz. bay leaf

- 1 teaspoon salt

- 1 teaspoon ground pepper

- 1 teaspoon coriander

- 4 oz. Feta cheese

Directions:

1. Put the chicken breast in the slow cooker.

2. Sprinkle the meat with the bay leaf, salt, ground pepper, and coriander.

3.   Add water and cook the chicken breast for 6 hours on LOW.

4.   Then remove the cooked chicken from the slow cooker and shred it with a fork.

5.   Chop the lettuce roughly.

6.   Then chop Feta cheese. Combine the chopped Ingredients: together and add the shredded chicken breast and Caesar dressing.

7.   Mix everything together well. After this, spread the tortillas with the shredded chicken mixture and wrap them. Enjoy!

Nutrition:

Calories 376,

Fat 18.5,

Fiber 3,

Carbs 29.43,

Protein 23

Dinner Recipes

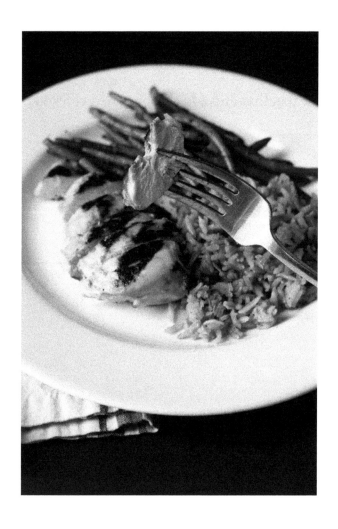

Pesto Shirataki Noodles–Vegan

Preparation time: 10 minutes

Cooking time: 7 minutes

Servings: 4

Ingredients

- Shirataki noodles (2–8-ounce packages)
- Fresh basil (2 cups packed)
- Minced garlic (1 clove)
- Pine nuts (.25 cup)
- Nutritional yeast (.25 cup)
- Salt (1 pinch)
- Olive or pistachio oil (.25 cup)

Directions:

1. Drain and rinse the shirataki noodles thoroughly. Boil for two to three minutes or microwave for one minute.

2. Combine the remainder of the fixings in a food processor, drizzling in olive oil while the motor is running.

3. Mix the pesto with the prepared noodles and serve.

Nutrition: Calories: 432 Fat: 22 g Carb: 2 g Protein: 21 g

Paleo Cabbage Slaw

Preparation time: 10 minutes

Cooking time: 15 minutes

Serves: 6

Ingredients:

- 1 cup Paleo Mayo (here)

- 2 to 3 tablespoons agave

- 2 tablespoons apple cider vinegar

- 2 teaspoons celery seed

- Salt

- Freshly ground black pepper

- 1 small to medium cabbage, spiralized

Directions:

1. In a small bowl, combine the mayonnaise, agave, apple cider vinegar, and celery seed. Stir well and season with salt and pepper.

2. In a large bowl, spoon the dressing over the cabbage noodles and toss to combine.

3. Refrigerate for at least 15 to 20 minutes before serving.

Nutrition: Calories 194 Fat 13g, Protein 11g, Carbs 2g, Fiber 21g

Salmon Pasta

Preparation time: 10 minutes

Cooking time: 7 minutes

Servings: 4

Ingredients

- Coconut oil (2 tablespoons)

- Smoked salmon (8 ounces)

- Zucchini (2)

- Keto-friendly mayo (.25 cup)

Directions:

1. Melt the oil in a skillet using the med-high temperature setting.

2. Add the salmon and sauté for 2-3 minutes or until lightly browned.

3. Prepare the zucchini using a peeler or spiralizer to make the noodle-like strands. Toss into the skillet and sauté for 1-2 minutes.

4. Mix in the mayo before serving.

Nutrition: Calories: 327 Fat: 21 g Carb: 3 g Protein: 21 g

Mushroom Pasta with Shirataki Noodles

Preparation time: 10 minutes

Cooking time: 20 minutes

Servings: 2

Ingredients

- Shirataki noodles (2 packages)

- Butter (2 tablespoons)

- Garlic (2 cloves)

- Assorted mushrooms (3 cups)

- Almond flour (1 teaspoon)

- Dried parsley (1 pinch)

- Thick cream (.75 of 1 tub)

- Salt (.25 teaspoon)

- Pepper (.25 teaspoon)

- Olive oil

- For the Garnish: Freshly chopped parsley

Directions:

1. Toss the shirataki noodles into a dry frying pan using the medium heat temperature setting. Continue to cook until

you hear a whistling sound, indicating the excess moisture leaving the noodles. Transfer to the countertop to cool.

2.   Toss the butter into the skillet with the garlic, and sauté for approximately 1 minute or until fragrant.

3.   Pour in the oil and add the mushrooms. Sauté for another five minutes, occasionally stirring until the mushrooms are golden in color. Transfer the mushrooms from the pan, leaving the oil behind.

4.   Add the almond flour, salt, pepper, dried parsley, and cream. Stir and simmer to combine.

5.   Lastly, toss the mushrooms and shirataki noodles into the skillet and combine. Serve right away.

Nutrition: Calories: 432 Fat: 22 g Carb: 2 g Protein: 21 g

Main

Chicken Noodle Soup Recipe

Preparation time: 5 minutes

Cooking Time: 30 minutes

Serving Size: 10

Ingredients:

- 1 tablespoon sea salt or to taste

- 1 garlic clove (pressed)

- 4 chicken thighs (skins removed)

- 3 tablespoon fresh dill

- 1 teaspoon salt-free seasoning

- 4 cups chicken broth

- 2 carrots (sliced)

- 1/2 lb. rotini pasta

- 10 cups water

- 2 medium celery sticks (finely chopped)

- 2 tablespoon olive oil

- 1 medium onion (finely chopped)

Directions:

1. Mix ten cups of water with four cups of chicken broth and one tablespoon of sea salt in a big soup pot.

2. Bring to a simmer, include chicken thighs and cook partly covered for twenty minutes while the vegetables are cooked, skimming off any bubble that floats on the surface.

3. Put two tablespoons of olive oil and sauté the onions and celery in a large skillet once soften, then switch to the bowl.

4. In the stockpot, 1/2 lb. of pasta and diced carrots and proceed to cook at a low simmer for fifteen minutes or until the pasta is tender.

5. Erase the chicken thighs from the container when cooking the pasta and use either tools or your fingers to slice the chicken, removing any bone and fat that can come off quickly.

6. Place the shredded chicken back in the pot.

7. Season with 1 teaspoon your preferred seasoning and if appropriate, additional salt to adjust.

8. Add one clove of garlic in the pan. Finally, insert three tablespoons of dill and extract it from the heat.

Nutrition: Calories: 213 Total Fat: 2g Carbs: 3g Protein: 9g

Savory Pine Nuts Cabbage

Preparation Time: 10 minutes Cooking Time: 2 hours

Servings: 2 Ingredients:

- 1 savoy cabbage, shredded

- 1 tablespoons of avocado oil

- 1 tablespoon of balsamic vinegar

- ¼ cup of pine nuts, toasted

- ½ cup of vegetable broth

Directions: Start by throwing all the ingredients into the Slow cooker. Cover its lid and cook for 2 hours on Low setting. Once done, remove its lid of the slow cooker carefully. Mix well and garnish as desired. Serve warm. Nutrition: Calories 145 Total Fat 13.1 g Saturated Fat 9.1 g Cholesterol 96 mg Sodium 35 mg Total Carbs 4 g Sugar 1.2 g Fiber 1.5 g Protein 3.5 g

Sardine Pate

Preparation time: 15 minutes

Cooking time: 3 hours

Servings: 6

Ingredients:

- ½ cup water

- 1 tablespoons butter

- 1 teaspoon onion powder

- 1 teaspoon dried parsley

- oz sardine fillets, chopped

Directions:

Put the chopped sardine fillets, dried parsley, onion powder, and water in the slow cooker.

Close the lid and cook the fish for 3 hours on Low.

Strain the sardine fillet and put it in a blender.

Add butter and blend the mixture for 3 minutes at high speed.

Transfer the cooked pate into serving bowls and serve!

Nutrition:

calories 170, fat 12.3, fiber 0, carbs 0.3,

protein 14.1

Classic Minestrone Soup

Preparation time: 5 minutes

Cooking Time: 1 hour 5 minutes

Serving Size: 6 bowls

Ingredients:

- 2 teaspoons lemon juice

- Fresh (grated) Parmesan cheese

- 4 tablespoons virgin olive oil (divided)

- 1 can beans

- 2 cups (chopped) collard greens

- 1 onion (chopped)

- (Freshly ground) black pepper

- 1 cup (whole grain) elbow or shell pasta

- 2 medium carrots (chopped)

- 2 ribs celery, (chopped)

- 2 bay leaves

- Pinch of red pepper flakes

- 1/3 cup tomato paste

- 2 cups (chopped) seasonal vegetables

- 2 cups of water

- 1 teaspoon fine sea salt

- 4 cloves garlic (minced)

- 1/2 teaspoon (dried) oregano

- 1 large can (diced) tomatoes

- 4 cups vegetable broth

- 1/2 teaspoon (dried) thyme

Directions:

1. Heat a skillet with oil.

2. Insert the sliced onions, cabbage, celery, tomato sauce and a touch of salt until the oil glitters.

3. Cook until the veggies are darkened, and the onions become translucent.

4. Seasonal tomatoes, ginger, oregano and chives can be added.

5. Cook until aromatic, for about two minutes, while whisking frequently.

6. Pour the sliced tomatoes, their liquids, broth, and water into the mixture.

7. Add lime, bay leaves and flakes of red pepper. With salt and black pepper, season generously.

8. Increase the heat to medium-high and put the mixture to a boil, then cover the pan with the lid partly, allowing a space of around one inch for steam to escape.

9. To sustain a gentle simmer, reduce the heat as needed.

10. Heat and remove the cap for fifteen minutes, then insert the spaghetti, beans and greens.

11. Continue to boil for twenty minutes, exposed, or until the pasta is prepared al dente and the vegetables are soft.

12. Erase the jar, then extract the bay leaves from the steam.

13. Add the lemon juice and the remaining tablespoon of essential oil and mix well.

14. Flavor it with more pepper and salt. Spice the soup bowls with parmesan cheese.

Nutrition: Calories: 111 Total Fat: 2g Carbs: 0g Protein: 9g

Spinach pasta

Preparation time: 2 minutes

Cooking time: 3 minutes

Serves: 5

Ingredients:

- 3 oz. spinach

- 2 eggs

- 1/2 tsp. salt

- 1 1/2 tsp. olive oil

- 2 cups almond flour

- 1/2 cup coconut flour, for kneading

Directions:

1.   Cook the spinach until it turns bright green.

2.   Prepare an ice bath for the spinach by combining ice and water in a large bowl.

3.   Remove the spinach from the skillet and submerge it in the ice water.

4.   Once the spinach is lukewarm, drain and squeeze the extra water with a cloth.

5.   Combine the spinach, eggs, salt, and olive oil in a bowl.

6.   Mix until everything is smooth.

7.   Slowly add the almond flour to make the dough.

8.   Once the dough is formed, let it sit for 25 minutes.

9.   Dust a flat workplace with a generous amount of coconut flour and knead the dough with it until the dough is no longer sticky. Add as needed.

10.   Cut the dough into 4 pieces.

11.   Roll each piece with a rolling pin.

12.   Using a pizza wheel, cut 3-4 inch blocks out of the dough.

13.   Cut the blocks in a zigzag motion to create medium sized triangles.

14.   Once all of them are cut, dust the triangles with some coconut flour.

15.   Take a piece of the triangle shaped pasta, wet your fingers and stick two of the ends together.

16.   Repeat with all of the triangle pieces.

17.   Lower the pasta gently in a pot of boiling water and cook for 3 minutes.

18.   Remove each piece and transfer to a plate.

Nutrition: Calories 165 Carbs 5 g Fiber 6 g Fat 17 g Protein 13.6 g

Cheese head lasagna sheets

Preparation time: 3 minutes

Cooking time: 15 minutes

Servings: 8

Ingredients:

- 1 egg

- 2 tbsps. cream cheese

- 3/4 cup almond flour

- 1 3/4 cups shredded mozzarella cheese

- 1/4 tsp. salt

- 1/2 tsp. Italian seasoning

Directions:

1. In a microwave safe bowl, mix the shredded cheese and almond flour.

2. Add the cream cheese on top of the mix.

3. Put the mix in the microwave for 30 seconds.

4. Mix in the Italian seasoning, salt, and egg.

5. Shape into a sphere with your hands.

6. Put the ball in in the middle of the two pieces of parchment paper.

7. Roll the dough out into a sheet using a rolling pin.

8. Remove the parchment paper on top.

9. Cut into 4 wide 6-inch-long pieces.

10. Prepare the lasagna sauce and filling.

11. Preheat the oven to 400F.

12. Cook for 12-15 minutes.

Nutrition: Calories: 275 Total Fat: 7.6g Carbs: 1.6g Protein: 6.3g

Spare Ribs

Preparation time: 10 minutes Cooking time: 8 hours

Servings: 6

Ingredients:

- 1-pound pork loin ribs

- 1 teaspoon olive oil

- 1 teaspoon minced garlic

- ¼ teaspoon cumin

- ¼ teaspoon chili powder

- 1 tablespoon butter

- 1 tablespoons water

Directions:

Mix the olive oil, minced garlic, cumin, and chili flakes in a bowl. Melt the butter and add to the spice mixture.

Stir it well and add water. Stir again.

Then rub the pork ribs with the spice mixture generously and place the ribs in the slow cooker. Close the lid and cook the ribs for 8 hours on Low. When the ribs are cooked, serve them immediately!

Nutrition: calories 203, fat 14.1, fiber 0.6, carbs 10, protein 9.8

Creamy Mustard Asparagus

Preparation Time: 10 minutes

Cooking Time: 3 hours

Servings: 2

Ingredients:

- 1 lb. asparagus, trimmed and halved

- 1 teaspoons of mustard

- ¼ cup of coconut cream

- garlic cloves, minced

- 1 tablespoon of chives, diced

- Salt and black pepper- to taste

Directions:

Start by throwing all the ingredients into the Slow cooker.

Cover its lid and cook for 3 hours on Low setting.

Once done, remove its lid of the slow cooker carefully.

Mix well and garnish as desired.

Serve warm.

Nutrition:

Calories 149

Total Fat 14.5 g

Saturated Fat 8.1 g

Cholesterol 56 mg

Sodium 56 mg

Total Carbs 10.6 g

Sugar 0.3 g

Fiber 0.2 g

Protein 2.6 g

Soups, Stews, and Chilis

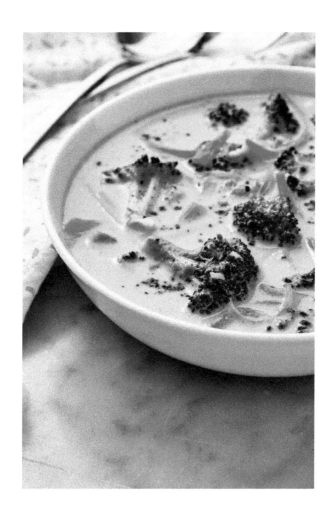

Broccoli Curry Soup

Preparation Time: 10 minutes

Cooking Time: 30 minutes

Servings: 4

Ingredients:

- Salt & Black pepper (as needed)
- Onion, chopped
- tbsp. Curry
- tbsp. Coconut oil
- liter Vegetable stock
- 1 cup Coconut cream
- 75 g Cheese substitute - your choice, grated
- 1 lb. Broccoli

Directions:

1. Pour coconut oil into a frying pan on the stovetop using the med-high heat setting.

2. Mix in the onion. Simmer for approximately six minutes.

3.   Lower the temperature to medium. Then, add in the broth until it begins to simmer. Mix in the broccoli as well as any seasonings before adding curry. Simmer for 20 minutes.

4.   Pour into a blender before mixing in the cheese substitute.

5.   well.

Nutrition: Calories: 375 Total, Fat Content: 20 g Net Carbs: 5 g Protein: 17 g

Easy Cheeseburger Casserole

Preparation Time: 10 minutes

Cooking time: 35 minutes

Servings: 5

Ingredients:

- cooking spray

Crust:

- 5 cups self-rising flour

- 3/4 cup sour cream

- 1 egg, beaten

- 1 cup water, or as needed

Topping:

- 2 pounds ground beef

- 1 onion, finely chopped

- 6 cups shredded Cheddar cheese

Directions:

1. Set the oven to 175°C (350°F). Spray cooking spray onto 3 round baking dishes.

2.   Combine the egg, sour cream, and flour with just a sufficient amount of water to bring the mixture into a spreadable consistency.

3.   Heat a big skillet on medium-high heat. Cook while stirring the onion and beef in the hot skillet for 5-7 minutes until the beef is completely browned. Strain and remove the grease. Put aside the beef mixture to cool.

4.   Split the dough mixture into 3 portions. Stretch each portion over the bottom of each prepared baking dish to cover. Spread approximately 1/3 the ground beef mixture onto each dough. Sprinkle approximately 2 cups of shredded Cheddar cheese on top of each. Use aluminum foil to cover each dish.

5.   Bake for 25-30 minutes in the preheated oven until the cheese bubbles and a bit browned.

Nutrition: calories 596, fat 16, carbs 33, protein 22

Vegetarian Fish Sauce

Preparation Time: 5 minutes

Cooking Time: 20 minutes

Servings: 16

Ingredients:

- 1/4 cup dried shiitake mushrooms

- 1-2 tbsp. tamari (for a depth of flavor)

- 3 tbsp. coconut aminos

- ¼ cup water

- tsp sea salt

Directions:

1. To a small saucepan, add water, coconut aminos, dried shiitake mushrooms, and sea salt. Bring to a boil, then cover, reduce heat, and simmer for 15-20 minutes.

2. Remove from heat and let cool slightly. Pour liquid through a fine-mesh strainer into a bowl, pressing on the mushroom mixture with a spoon to squeeze out any remaining liquid.

3.   To the bowl, add tamari. Taste and adjust as needed, adding more sea salt for saltiness.

4.   Store in a sealed container in the refrigerator for up to 1 month and shake well before use. Or pour into an ice cube tray, freeze, and store in a freezer-safe container for up to 2 months.

Nutrition: Calories: 39.1 Fat: 2g Carbs: 5g Protein: 0.3g

Black Bean Mushroom Chili

Preparation Time: 17 minutes Cooking time: 8 hours 25

Minutes

Servings: 10

Ingredients:

- 2 1/2 cups black beans, rinsed and drained

- 1 tbsp. olive oil

- 2 tbsp. chili powder

- 1/4 cup mustard seeds

- 1/2 tsp. cardamom seeds

- 1 1/2 tsp. cumin seeds

- 1/4 cup water

- 1 lb. mushrooms, sliced

- 2 onions, chopped

- 5 cups vegetable stock

- 1 tbsp. chipotle pepper in adobo sauce, chopped

- 6 oz. tomato paste

- 1 cup cheddar cheese, grated

- 1/2 cup sour cream

- 1/2 fresh cilantro, chopped

Directions:

1.   Soak black beans overnight. Rinse and drain the next day.

2.   Place oil, chili powder, mustard, cardamom, and cumin in a Dutch oven.

3.   Cook over high heat for 30 seconds.

4.   Add water, mushrooms, and onions.

5.   Cover and cook for 7 minutes. Add broth, chipotles, and tomato paste.

6.   Cook for another 15 minutes.

7.   Put the beans in a slow cooker.

8.   Add the vegetable mixture. Cook on high for 8 hours.

9.   Garnish with sour cream, cilantro, and cheese before serving. Enjoy!

Nutrition: calories 216, fat 10, carbs 13, protein 10

Tomato Bisque Soup

Preparation time: 10 minutes

Cooking time: 40 minutes

Servings: 6

Ingredients:

- 3 cups canned whole, peeled tomatoes
- 4 cups chicken broth
- cup heavy cream
- cloves garlic, chopped
- tablespoons butter
- teaspoon freshly chopped thyme
- Salt & black pepper, to taste

Directions:

1. Add the butter to the bottom of a stockpot.

2. Add in all the remaining ingredients minus the heavy cream. Bring to a boil, and then simmer for 40 minutes.

3. Warm the heavy cream, and then stir into the soup.

Nutrition: Calories: 144 Carbs: 4g Fiber: 1g Net Carbs: 3g Fat: 12g Protein: 4g

Swedish Pea and Ham Soup

Preparation Time: 10 minutes

Cooking time: 5 hours

Servings: 8

Ingredients:

- 3 cups yellow split peas, rinsed and drained

- 4 cups water

- 4 cups low sodium chicken stock

- 1 cup carrots, diced

- 2 cups onions, diced

- 1 tbsp. fresh ginger, minced

- 8 oz. ham, sliced

- 1 tsp. dried marjoram

- 1/4 tsp. pepper

Directions:

1. Put the split peas, water, stock, carrots, onions, celery, ginger, ham, and marjoram in the slow cooker.

2. Stir to blend everything. Put the lid on.

3. Cook on high for 4 ½ to 5 hours.

4. Season with pepper before serving. Enjoy!

Nutrition: calories 338, fat 3, carbs 23, protein 21

Broccoli Cheddar & Bacon Soup

Preparation time: 10 minutes

Cooking time: 10 minutes

Servings: 6

Ingredients:

- 2 cups chicken broth

- cup broccoli florets finely chopped

- cup heavy cream

- cup shredded cheddar cheese

- ½ white onion, chopped

- cloves garlic, chopped

- slices cooked bacon, crumbled for serving

- ½ teaspoon salt

- ¼ teaspoon black pepper

Directions:

1. Add all the ingredients minus the heavy cream, cheddar cheese and bacon to a stockpot over medium heat.

2. Bring to a simmer and cook for 5 minutes.

3.   Warm the cream, and then add the warm cream and cheddar cheese. Whisk until smooth.

4.   Serve with crumbled bacon.

Nutrition: Calories: 220 Carbs: 4g Fiber: 1g Net Carbs: 3g Fat: 18g Protein: 11g

Fish and Seafood

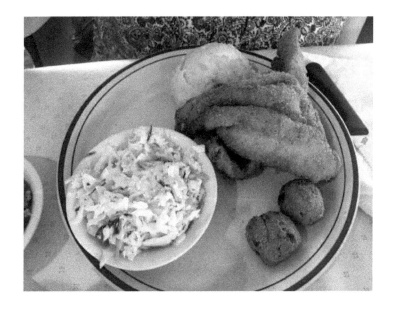

Oregano Salmon

Preparation Time: 15 minutes   Cooking time: 1 hour 30 minutes   Servings: 2

Ingredients:

- 2 salmon steaks (2 fillets 6 oz each)
- 1 tablespoon oregano, dried
- 1 teaspoon smoked paprika
- 2 tablespoons olive oil
- 6 tablespoons water
- ½ teaspoon salt
- ½ teaspoon balsamic vinegar

Directions:

1.   In the slow cooker, mix the salmon with the oregano and the other ingredients.

2.   Close the lid and cook salmon for 1.5 hours on High.

Nutrition: calories 223, fat 12, carbs 5, protein 14

Crab Dip

Preparation Time: 15 minutes   Cooking time: 2 hours

Servings: 3   Ingredients:

- 1 cup crabmeat
- 1 cup Cheddar cheese, shredded
- ½ cup of coconut milk
- 2 spring onions, chopped
- 1 teaspoon olive oil
- 1 teaspoon paprika
- 1 teaspoon oregano, dried
- ½ teaspoon salt
- ½ teaspoon dried cilantro

Directions:

1.   In the slow cooker, mix the crabmeat with the cheese and the other ingredients and whisk.

2.   Close the lid and cook the dip for 2 hours on High.

3.   Mix up it well with the help of the spoon.

Nutrition: calories 310, fat 13, carbs 5, protein 22

Ginger Mackerel

Preparation Time: 15 minutes   Cooking time: 1 hour 30 minutes Servings: 6 Ingredients:

- 2-pound mackerel
- 1 teaspoon fresh ginger, minced
- 1 teaspoon ground cumin
- 1 teaspoon salt
- 1 teaspoon black pepper
- 1 teaspoon turmeric powder
- 1 teaspoon lemon juice
- ½ teaspoon lemon rind, grated
- ½ cup of coconut milk
- 1 teaspoon coconut oil

Directions: In the slow cooker, mix the mackerel with the ginger, cumin, and the other ingredients. Close the slow cooker lid and cook fish for 1.5 hours on High. Divide between plates and serve.

Nutrition: calories 321, fat 9, carbs 3, protein 20

Vegetable

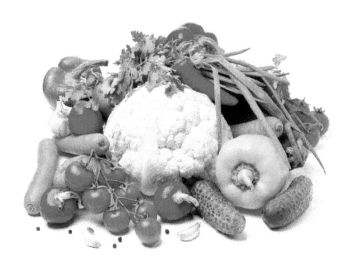

Zucchini Balls

Preparation time: 20 minutes

Cooking time: 30 minutes

Servings: 4

Ingredients

- 1 cup zucchini, grated
- ½ cup almond flour
- ¼ cup Parmesan, grated
- 1 egg, whisked
- 1 tablespoon avocado oil
- ¾ cup of coconut milk
- ½ teaspoon salt

Directions:

1. In the mixing bowl zucchinis with flour and the other Ingredients: except the coconut milk and the oil and shape medium balls.

2. Preheat avocado oil in the skillet and add zucchini balls.

3. Roast them for 2 minutes from each side.

4. After this, transfer the zucchini balls in the slow cooker. Add coconut milk and close the lid.

5.   Cook the meal for 30 minutes on High.

Nutrition : calories 207, fat 5.5, fibre 1.8, carbs 4.5, protein 3.6

Butter Green Peas

Preparation time: 10 minutes

Cooking time: 3 hours

Servings: 4

Ingredients

- 1 cup green peas

- 1 teaspoon minced garlic

- 1 tablespoon butter, softened

- ½ teaspoon cayenne pepper

- 1 tablespoon olive oil

- ¾ teaspoon salt

- 1 teaspoon paprika

- 1 teaspoon garam masala

- ½ cup chicken stock

Directions:

1. In the slow cooker, mix the peas with butter, garlic and the other Ingredients:,

2. Close the lid and cook for 3 hours on High.

Nutrition: calories 121, fat 6.5, fiber 3, carbs 3.4, protein 0.6

Lemon Asparagus

Preparation time: 8 minutes

Cooking time: 5 hours

Servings: 2

Ingredients

- 8 oz. asparagus

- ½ cup butter

- juice of 1 lemon

- Zest of 1 lemon, grated

- ½ teaspoon turmeric

- 1 teaspoon rosemary, dried

Directions:

1.	In your slow cooker, mix the asparagus with butter, lemon juice and the other Ingredients: and close the lid.

2.	Cook the vegetables on Low for 5 hours. Divide between plates and serve.

Nutrition: calories 139, fat 4.6., fiber 2.5, carbs 3.3, protein 3.5

Curry Cauliflower

Preparation time: 15 minutes

Cooking time: 2.5 hours

Servings: 4

Ingredients

- 1 ½ cup cauliflower, trimmed and florets separated

- 1 tablespoon curry paste

- ½ cup coconut cream

- 1 teaspoon butter

- ½ teaspoon garam masala

- ¾ cup chives, chopped

- 1 tablespoon rosemary, chopped

- 2 tablespoons Parmesan, grated

Directions:

1. In the slow cooker, mix the cauliflower with the curry paste and the other Ingredients.

2. Cook the cauliflower for 2.5 hours on High.

Nutrition: calories 146, fat 4.3, fiber 1.9, carbs 5.7, protein 5.3

Creamy Broccoli

Preparation time: 15 minutes

Cooking time: 1 hour

Servings: 4

Ingredients

- ½ cup coconut cream

- 2 cups broccoli florets

- 1 teaspoon mint, dried

- 1 teaspoon garam masala

- 1 teaspoon salt

- 1 tablespoon almonds flakes

- ½ teaspoon turmeric

Directions:

1. In the slow cooker, mix the broccoli with the mint and the other Ingredients.

2. Close the lid and cook vegetables for 1 hour on High.

3. Divide between plates and serve.

Nutrition: calories 102, fat 9, fiber 1.9, carbs 4.3, protein 2.5

Meat

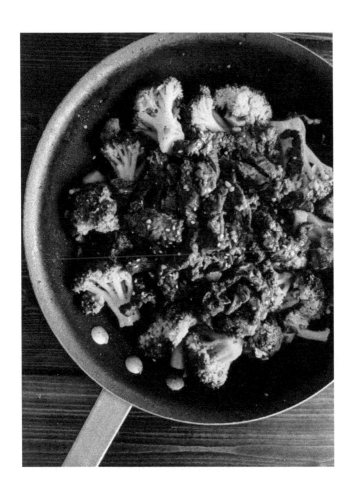

Kalua Pork with Cabbage

Preparation time: 10 minutes Cooking time: 9 hours

Servings: 12

Ingredients

*   1 medium cabbage head, chopped

*   1 lbs. pork shoulder butt roast, trimmed

*   bacon slices

*   1 tbsp. sea salt

Directions:

*   Place 4 bacon slices into the bottom of the slow cooker. Spread pork roast on top of bacon slices and season with salt. Arrange remaining bacon slices on top of the pork roast layer. Cover slow cooker with lid and cook on low for8 hours or until meat is tender. Add chopped cabbage. Cover again and cook on low for 1 hour. Remove pork from the slow cooker and shred using a fork. Return shredded pork to the slow cooker and stir well. Serve warm and enjoy.

Nutrition: Calories 264 Fat 18.4 g Carbohydrates 4.4 g Sugar 2.4 g Protein 20.5 g Cholesterol 71 mg

Braised Beef Strips

Preparation time: 10 minutes

Cooking time: 5 hours

Servings: 4

Ingredients

- ½ cup mushroom, sliced

- 1 onion, sliced

- 1 cup of water

- 1 tablespoon coconut oil

- 1 teaspoon salt

- 1 teaspoon white pepper

- oz. beef loin, cut into strips

Directions

1   Melt the coconut oil in the skillet.

2   Add mushrooms and roast them for 5 minutes on medium heat.

3   Then transfer the mushrooms to the slow cooker.

4   Add all remaining Ingredients: and close the lid.

5   Cook the meal on High for 5 hours

Nutrition:

173 calories,

19.6g protein,

3.2g carbohydrates,

9.4g fat,

0.8g fiber,

50mg cholesterol,

624mg sodium,

316mg potassium

Creamy Pork Chops

Preparation time: 10 minutes

Cooking time: 6 hours

Servings: 4

Ingredients

- boneless pork chops
- ½ cup chicken stock
- 1 oz. dry ranch dressing
- oz. chicken soup
- garlic cloves, minced
- Pepper

Directions:

1   Season pork chops with pepper and place in a slow cooker. In a bowl, mix together chicken soup, ranch dressing, stock, and garlic. Pour chicken soup mixture over top of pork chops. Cover slow cooker with lid and cook on low for 6 hours. Serve hot and enjoy.

Nutrition: Calories 280 Fat 15.1 g Carbohydrates 7.4 g Sugar 1 g Protein 29.1 g Cholesterol 64 mg

Side Dish Recipes

Cabbage and Onion Mix

Preparation time: 15 minutes

Cooking time: 2 Hours

Servings: 2

Ingredients

- 1 and ½ cups green cabbage, shredded

- 1 cup red cabbage, shredded

- 1 tablespoon olive oil

- 1 red onion, sliced

- 2 spring onions, chopped

- ½ cup tomato paste

- ¼ cup veggie stock

- 2 tomatoes, chopped

- 2 jalapenos, chopped

- 1 tablespoon chili powder

- 1 tablespoon chives, chopped

- A pinch of salt and black pepper

Directions:

1.   Grease your Crock Pot with the oil and mix the cabbage with the onion, spring onions and the other Ingredients: inside.

2.   Toss, put the lid on and cook on High for hours.

3.   Divide between plates and serve as a side dish.

Nutrition: calories 211, fat 3, fiber 3, carbs 6, protein 8

Cauliflower and Potatoes Mix

Preparation time: 15 minutes

Cooking time: 4 Hours

Servings: 2

Ingredients

- 1 cup cauliflower florets
- ½ pound sweet potatoes, peeled and cubed
- 1 cup veggie stock
- ½ cup tomato sauce
- 1 tablespoon chives, chopped
- Salt and black pepper to the taste
- 1 teaspoon sweet paprika

Directions:

1. In your Crock Pot, mix the cauliflower with the potatoes, stock and the other Ingredients, toss, put the lid on and cook on High for 4 hours.

2. Divide between plates and serve as a side dish.

Nutrition: calories 135, fat 5, fiber 1, carbs 7, protein 3

Cumin Quinoa Pilaf

Preparation time: 15 minutes

Cooking time: 2 Hours

Servings: 2

Ingredients

- 1 cup quinoa
- 2 teaspoons butter, melted
- Salt and black pepper to the taste
- 1 teaspoon turmeric powder
- 2 cups chicken stock
- 1 teaspoon cumin, ground

Directions:

1. Grease your Crock Pot with the butter, add the quinoa and the other Ingredients:, toss, put the lid on and then cook on High for about 2 hours

2. Divide between plates and serve as a side dish.

Nutrition: calories 152, fat 3, fiber 6, carbs 8, protein 4

Cauliflower Rice and Spinach

Preparation time: 15 minutes

Cooking time: 3 Hours

Servings: 8

Ingredients

- 2 garlic cloves, minced
- 2 tablespoons butter, melted
- 1 yellow onion, chopped
- ¼ teaspoon thyme, dried
- 3 cups veggie stock
- 20 ounces spinach, chopped
- 6 ounces coconut cream
- Salt and black pepper to the taste
- 2 cups cauliflower rice

Directions:

1. Heat up a pan with the butter over medium heat, add onion, stir and cook for 4 minutes.

2. Add garlic, thyme and stock, stir, cook for 1 minute more and transfer to your Crock Pot.

3. Add spinach, coconut cream, cauliflower rice, salt and pepper, stir a bit, cover and cook on High for hours.

4. Divide between plates and serve as a side dish.

—

Nutrition: calories 200, fat 4, fibre 4, carbs 8, protein 2

Appetizers & Snacks

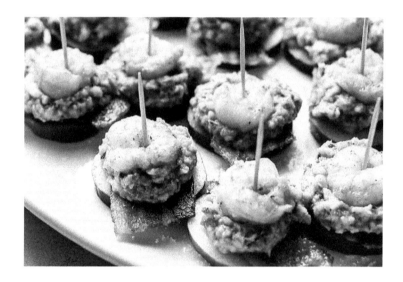

Butter Asparagus with Creamy Eggs

Preparation time: 5 minutes

Cooking time: 8 minutes

Servings: 2

Ingredients:

- 4 oz asparagus

- 2 eggs, blended

o   oz grated parmesan cheese

- 1-ounce sour cream

- 2 tbsp butter, unsalted

- Seasoning:

- 1/3 tsp salt

- 1/8 tsp ground black pepper

- ¼ tsp cayenne pepper

- ½ tbsp avocado oil

Directions:

1.   Take a medium skillet pan, place it over medium heat, add butter and when it melts, add blended eggs and then cook for 2 to 3 minutes until scrambled to the desired level; don't overcook.

2.	Spoon the scrambled eggs into a food processor, add 1/8 tsp salt, cayenne pepper, sour cream and cheese and then pulse for 1 minute until smooth.

3.	Return skillet pan over medium heat, add oil and when hot, add asparagus, season with black pepper and remaining salt, toss until mixed and cook for 3 minutes or more until roasted.

4.	Distribute asparagus between two plates, add egg mixture, and then serve.

Nutrition: 338 Calories; 28.5 g Fats; 14.4 g Protein; 4.7 g Net Carb; 1.2 g Fiber;

Turkey and Cabbage Treat

Preparation Time: 5 minutes

Cooking time: 5 minutes

Servings: 4

Ingredients:

- tablespoon lard, at room temperature

- 1/2 cup onion, chopped

- pound ground turkey

- 10 ounces puréed tomatoes

- Sea salt and ground black pepper, to taste

- teaspoon cayenne pepper

- 1/4 teaspoon caraway seeds

- 1/4 teaspoon mustard seeds

- 1/2 pound cabbage, cut into wedges

- 4 garlic cloves, minced

- 1 cup chicken broth

- bay leaves

Directions:

1. Press the "Sauté" button to heat up your Instant Pot. Then, melt the lard. Cook the onion until translucent and tender.

2. Add ground turkey and cook until it is no longer pink; reserve the turkey/onion mixture.

3. Mix puréed tomatoes with salt, black pepper, cayenne pepper, caraway seeds, and mustard seeds.

4. Spritz the bottom and sides of the Instant Pot with a nonstick cooking spray. Then, place 1/2 of cabbage wedges on the bottom of your Instant Pot.

5. Spread the meat mixture over the top of the cabbage. Add minced garlic. Add the remaining cabbage.

6. Now, pour in the tomato mixture and chicken broth; lastly, add bay leaves.

7. Secure the lid. Choose "Manual" mode and High pressure; cook for 5 minutes. Once cooking is complete, use a natural pressure release; carefully remove the lid.Bon appétit!

Nutrition: 247 Calories; 12.5g Fat; 6.2g Total Carbs; 25.3g Protein; 3.7g Sugars

Spinach Egg Muffins

Preparation time: 5 minutes

Cooking time: 10 minutes

Servings: 2

Ingredients:

- ½ cups chopped spinach

- 1/8 tsp dried basil

- 1/8 tsp garlic powder

- 2 large eggs

- 3 tbsp grated Parmesan cheese

- Seasoning:

- ¼ tsp of sea salt

- 1/8 tsp ground black pepper

Directions:

1. Turn on the oven, then set it to 400 degrees F, and let preheat.

2. Meanwhile, place eggs in a bowl, season with salt and black pepper and whisk until blended.

3. Add garlic and basil, whisk in mixed and then stir in spinach and cheese until combined.

4.   Take two silicone muffin cups, grease them with reserved bacon greased, fill them evenly with prepared egg mixture and bake for 8 to 10 minutes until the top has nicely browned.

5.   Serve.

Nutrition: 55 Calories; 3.5 g Fats; 4.5 g Protein; 0.4 g Net Carb; 0.2 g Fiber;

Broccoli and Egg Muffin

Preparation time: 10 minutes

Cooking time: 10 minutes

Servings: 2

Ingredients:

- ¼ cup broccoli florets, steamed, chopped

- 2 tbsp grated cheddar cheese

- 1/16 tsp dried thyme

- 1/16 tsp garlic powder

- egg

- Seasoning:

- ¼ tsp salt

- 1/8 tsp ground black pepper

Directions:

1. Turn on the oven, then set it to 400 degrees F and let it preheat.

2. Meanwhile, take two silicone muffin cups, grease them with oil, and evenly fill them with broccoli and cheese.

3.   Crack the egg in a bowl, add garlic powder, thyme, salt, and black pepper, whisk well, then evenly pour the mixture into muffin cups and bake for 8 to 10 minutes until done.

4.   Serve.

Nutrition: 76 Calories; 5.1 g Fats; 5.7 g Protein; 1.2 g Net Carb; 0.7 g Fiber;

Amazing Carrots Side Dish

Preparation time: 10 minutes

Cooking time: 10 minutes

Servings: 12

Ingredients:

- 3 pounds carrots, peeled and cut into medium pieces
- A pinch of sea salt and black pepper
- ½ cup water
- ½ cup maple syrup
- 2 tablespoons olive oil
- ½ teaspoon orange rind, grated

Directions:

1. Put the oil in your instant pot, add the carrots and toss.

2. Add maple syrup, water, salt, pepper and orange rind, stir, cover and cook on High for 10 minutes.

3. Divide among plates and serve as a side dish.

4. Enjoy!

Nutrition: Calories 140, fat 2, fiber 1, carbs 2, protein 6

Acorn Squash Puree

Preparation Time: 10 minutes

Cooking Time: 20 minutes

Servings: 4

Ingredients:

- ½ cup water
- 2 acorn squash, deseeded and halved
- Salt and black pepper to the taste
- 2 tablespoons ghee, melted
- ½ teaspoon nutmeg, grated

Directions:

1. Put the squash halves and the water in a pot, bring to a simmer, cook for 20 minutes, drain, scrape squash flesh, transfer to a bowl, add salt, pepper, ghee and nutmeg, mash well, divide between plates and serve as a side dish.

Nutrition: Calories: 182 Fat: 3 Fiber: 2 Carbs: 7 Protein: 6

Desserts

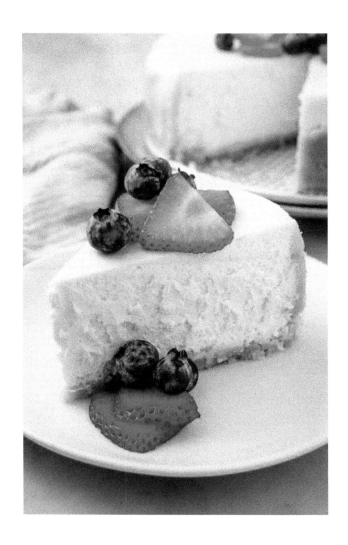

Rich Flavor Grain-Free Brownies

Preparation Time: 10 minutes

Cooking time: 4 hours

Servings: 12

Ingredients:

- ¼ cup unsalted butter, plus more for coating the slow cooker insert
- 4 ounces unsweetened chocolate, chopped
- Flour
- Cocoa powder
- ¼ cup coconut flour
- Salt
- 1 large ripe avocado, peeled, pitted, and mashed
- ¼ cup heavy (whipping) cream
- Eggs
- ¾ cup erythritol
- ¾ teaspoon stevia powder
- ¾ cup coarsely chopped walnuts

Directions:

1.   Coat the bottom and sides of the slow cooker insert with butter, then line the bottom with parchment or wax paper (trace the bottom of the insert on the parchment and then cut it out).

2.   In a small, microwave-safe bowl, combine ¼ cup of butter and the chocolate. Heat for 30-second intervals on high, stirring after each interval, until the chocolate is melted and the ingredients are fully incorporated.

3.   In a medium bowl, stir together the almond flour, cocoa powder, coconut flour, baking powder, and salt. In a large bowl, mix the avocado and heavy cream until smooth.

4.   Add the eggs, erythritol, and stevia and mix to combine. Mix in the melted chocolate until incorporated.

5.   Add the dry ingredients to the wet ingredients and mix until incorporated. Stir in the walnuts.

6.   Transfer the mixture to the slow cooker and spread evenly. Cover and cook for 4 hours on low. Let cool for about 30 minutes in the slow cooker. Run a knife around the edge and then lift out of the insert. Cut into pieces and serve at room temperature.

Nutrition: calories 229, fat 21, carbs 8, protein 10

Coconut Toasted Almond Cheesecake

Preparation Time: 10 minutes

Cooking time: 4 hours

Servings: 8

Ingredients:

FOR THE CRUST

- 1 cup toasted almonds, ground to a meal

- 1 large egg, lightly beaten

- 2 tablespoons coconut oil, melted

- 1 teaspoon stevia powder

- 1 cup water

FOR THE FILLING

- 2 large eggs

- 2 (8-ounce) packages cream cheese, at room temperature

- ¾ cup almond butter

- ¼ cup coconut cream

- 1 teaspoon pure almond extract

- ¾ cup erythritol

- 1 tablespoon coconut flour

- 2 teaspoons stevia powder

Directions:

TO MAKE THE CRUST

1. In a medium bowl, mix the almond meal, egg, coconut oil, and stevia powder.

2. Press the mixture into the bottom of a baking pan that fits into your slow cooker (make sure there is room to lift the pan out). Many pans could work, depending on the size and shape of your slow cooker.

3. Pour the water into the slow cooker insert. Place the pan in the cooker.

TO MAKE THE FILLING

1. In a large bowl, beat the eggs, then beat in the cream cheese, almond butter, coconut cream, almond extract, erythritol, coconut flour, and stevia powder. Pour the mixture over the crust. Cover and cook for 4 hours on low or 2 hours on high.

2. When finished, turn off the slow cooker and let the cheesecake sit inside until cooled to room temperature, up to 3 hours.

3.   Remove the pan from the slow cooker and refrigerate until chilled, about 2 hours more. Serve chilled.

Nutrition: calories 538, fat 5, carbs 13, protein 14

Lightning Source UK Ltd.
Milton Keynes UK
UKHW020750030621
384855UK00001B/53